To: Ben

Caged Bird
BY MAYA ANGELOU
A free bird leaps
on the back of the wind
and floats downstream
till the current ends

and dips his wing
in the orange sun rays
and dares to claim the sky.

But a bird that stalks
down his narrow cage
can seldom see through
his bars of rage
his wings are clipped and
his feet are tied
so, he opens his throat to sing.

The caged bird sings
with a fearful trill
of things unknown
but longed for still
and his tune is heard
on the distant hill
for the caged bird
sings of freedom.

The free bird thinks of another breeze
and the trade winds soft through the sighing trees
and the fat worms waiting on a dawn bright lawn
and he names the sky his own

But a caged bird stands on the grave of dreams
his shadow shouts on a nightmare scream
his wings are clipped and his feet are tied
so, he opens his throat to sing.

The caged bird sings
with a fearful trill
of things unknown
but longed for still
and his tune is heard
on the distant hill
for the caged bird

sings of freedom.

My Life After Agoraphobia,
What Now?

My Life After Agoraphobia, What Now?

YOLANDA ANTONINO

ISBN-13: 9781540300942
ISBN-10: 1540300943

IT HAS BEEN about 9 years since I found my way out of the rabbit hole of Agoraphobia. In 2014 I wrote a book "MY SILENT DISABILITY" by the same author, and told how my agoraphobia came about and how it impacted my life and my family's life. I thought it was time to tell you what my life has been like since most of my agoraphobic symptoms have left.

I have a condition called Vertical Heterophoria. Sounds bad, doesn't it? This is a condition of the eyes. There are over 1.8 million Americans 18 and over who suffer from Agoraphobia. There are no figures for Vertical Heterophoria because no one knows about it, much less how to treat it. But actually, there are 1.8 million with Vertical Heterophoria also. If you have one you have the other. THAT IS THE CAUSE OF AGORAPHOBIA. There are also people who have this condition because of traumatic brain injury and epilepsy.

Vertical Heterophoria is a condition where one eye focuses higher than the other. It is a form of Binocular Vision Dysfunction (BVD). In BVD, the two eyes have difficulty working together as a team. That is because one eye is aimed slightly higher than the other eye. Don't rush out to find the nearest optometrist office near you because they can't help you. They will pass a spoon like thing across your eyes and tell you, you are fine. They just weren't taught in school how to find Vertical Heterophoria. Most people with VH have 20/20 vision.

I found my condition myself by believing that I was not mentally ill and something was going on that I could not control. I was twenty-eight when my agoraphobia revealed itself. After pretty much giving up hope that I would ever find the answer it happened! One day while I was in the shower, after turning around really quick, my eyes did something funny. Now at this time I had agoraphobia for over 40 years and never had anything like this happen.

Before stepping into the shower, I had had a major panic attack so maybe that had something to do with it. I was new to the computer but after the shower I ran to it and looked up (eyes and agoraphobia). There it was, a whole site talking about this subject and a test to take to see if I was a candidate for this. I took the test and found out that, yes, I definitely was. There was just one problem. The doctor was in Michigan and I was in Illinois. This was going to be a big leap of faith getting there. Now I had to spend time on the road and time in a hotel and time in restaurants, all things that were triggers to my panic attacks. But I was convinced that I indeed had this condition, so I left my safe place and my husband drove me to Michigan. That started a wild journey of 3 years of pulling myself out of the bottom and working my way to the top. I am actually still improving after 9 years. I will tell you how you can do this also.

This is what is actually happening to your eyes and causing your symptoms:

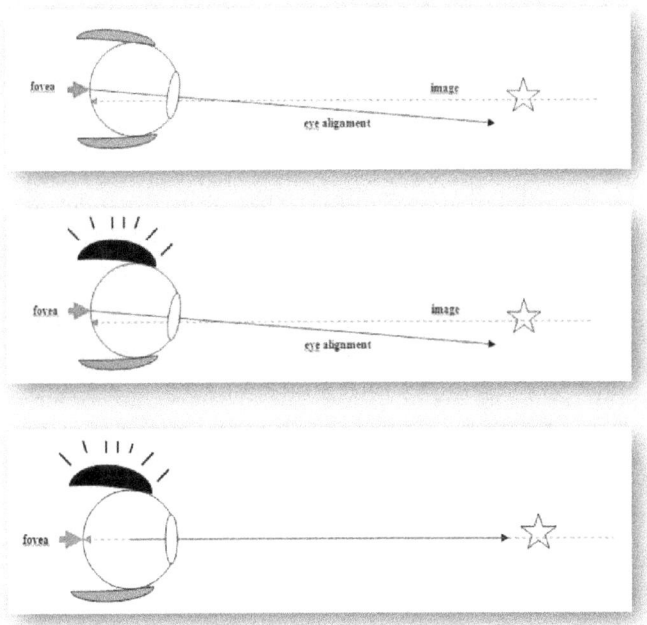

In the top picture the eye is looking down. It is not in alignment with the star.

In the second picture the eye muscles strain to correct the misalignment, after much struggle it now aligns with the star. Most people can depend on their eye muscles to correct this problem to a certain extant but eventually the muscles get tired and start to give out. It usually takes a traumatic event to totally give out. Or stress over a long period. As we get older and stress starts to take over we start to have symptoms. Some babies have symptoms out of the womb. More and more this is showing up in younger people, even in grade school. I was 28 years old with two children when mine hit. Sometimes the symptoms come and go. You seem to be doing fine for a year or so and then when some problem hits you start to feel dizzy, or anxious, or afraid and don't know why. The struggle of the eye to right itself causes the eye to quiver and that quivering brings on the dizziness. This dizziness in itself is strange. It's like sitting in a car in a parking lot and the car next to yours starts to move and you are not sure if it is you moving or the other car. Even though you are still, you feel like you are moving. Eyes that are misaligned cause blurred or double vision. The brain does not tolerate blurred or double vision, so it forces the eyes to look at the exact same spot, so that only one image is seen This is accomplished by straining the eye muscles to make one eye look up a little more, and the other eye to look down a little more. As the muscles strain, they become fatigued and jittery, and can no longer keep the eyes in the correct alignment. This "bouncing" in and out of alignment creates the feeling of dizziness, lightheaded, vertigo and a sense of imbalance. Like the situation of the car in the parking lot.

Agoraphobia is defined as "Fear of open Space." A better definition would be "Inability to define spatial awareness."

They both have to do with space but my definition describes it more accurately. Spatial awareness is being able to understand your body and how it fits in space. Most people don't think about this concept. It's an automatic response. They don't stop before going through the door to see if they are going to hit the side. But once agoraphobia hits this is not the case. We don't like open space because there are no anchors for our eyes to keep us grounded so we have that floating feeling. Balance depends on information received by the brain from three peripheral sources. EYES, MUSCLES AND JOINTS and VESTIBULAR ORGANS. As we saw before, our eyes are not focusing properly because of BVD so it makes perfect sense why we are experiencing these symptoms. We do much better in small spaces with lots of things around, this makes it easy for our eyes to find something to ground us.

What happens to you when all of this starts? You retreat when the fight or flight response takes over. YOU ARE UNDER ATTACK! The threat to your survival is real. Can you understand now why you can't come out of the bedroom? It's like the soldier in the trenches, he is not leaving the trench until the all clear is called. The problem is this, there is never an all clear for the agoraphobic, they're always under attack. Sometimes all symptoms go away for a while only to come back with a vengeance when a stressful time in your life happens. The fear of this happening again forces the agoraphobic into their house. It becomes their safe place. If you could think of this as a bomb attack everyone would be in a safe place. The feelings are very real. This is not your imagination dreaming this all up. The older you get the harder it is for the muscles to keep the eyes aligned. By now I'm sure you have a few questions like, WHAT, how did this happen to me? Does this happen to everyone?

It is definitely an "ALL IN THE FAMILY" disability. You might have had an Aunt Genevieve or an Uncle Joe that were a bit strange. This could have been their problem. Some cases of this condition may be caused by head trauma, stroke, or neurological disorders. Maybe some who have had a few symptoms of agoraphobia have had a car accident or fell and this put them in full force agoraphobia. Maybe you played football as a child or adult and a hit to the head caused this. Also, soldiers have come home with this condition. It's called TBI or traumatic brain injury. The eye muscles become jarred and misaligned. In my family, we have Diabetes and BVD. More women than men have agoraphobia I am not sure why.

Are you starting to understand now why you get overwhelmed or anxious in crowds or with driving? Some people have face pain, eye pain, TMJ problems, neck ache and upper back pain due to a head tilt. The head tilt is the body's way of trying to align the eyes. Look at pictures of yourself and see if your head is tilted to the side. I realize that a lot of us tilt our head in a picture but not in every one and not to the severe angle you will see. My head was so tilted it was almost flat. You might get motion sickness, nausea, poor depth perception unsteadiness while walking or drifting to one side while walking. Lack of coordination similar to those see in patients with MS, or stroke, and inner ear disorder or Meniere's Disease. Maybe you have reading symptoms such as difficulty with reading and comprehension, skipping lines while reading, losing one's place while reading, words running together while reading, similar to those seen with a learning disability. This can also cause ATTENTION DEFICIT DISORDER. You might have blurred vision, double or overlapping vision, shadowed vision, light sensitivity, difficulty with glare or reflection. Psychological symptom such as feeling overwhelmed or anxious when in large contained spaces like malls or big box stores like Wal-Mart. Feeling overwhelmed or anxious in crowds or when driving. Chronic migraines are also a part of this. Thanks to the internet this information is available to everyone. The internet is God's gift to mankind. That is where I went when all else failed.

The pioneer in this field is an eye doctor in Michigan. Her name is Dr. Debby Feinberg and she is at VISION SPECIALISTS OF MICHIGAN. There are a handful of other doctors that Dr. Debby has taught to find BVD= BINOCULAR VISION DYSFUNCTION and treat it. Later on, I will list those doctors. Since this concept is not taught in optometry school and BVD is not very well understood it was unlikely that anyone would come up with this information.

Here is the story of how Dr. Debby Feinberg stumbled upon the reason why agoraphobia happens:

In 1985 Dr. Debby was on a double date with the man who eventually would become her husband and his brother. While they were driving, she noticed Arthur her husband's brother, holding a large hand-held prism up to one of his eyes. She asked him what he was doing with it. He explained that he had been having eye strain issues, and had seen the chief of Ophthalmology at his medical school. He had a thorough eye exam, yet nothing was found amiss. Arthur maintained that there must be something wrong, as he could feel the strain, and the doctor gave him the hand-held prism, with the instructions to exercise his eyes with it to see if he could reduce the feelings of strain. Dr. Debby asked him if it helped but he said not much. She said he should come in to the office for an eye exam, and if he really needed a prismatic correction, she could make it part of his prescription in his lenses and he could wear it full-time. It turned out he needed vertical prismatic correction and he became her first Heterophoria (VH) patient. And so the die was cast for the cure of 1.8 million agoraphobics. If only they could be reached and convinced this was their problem. But the story didn't end there. It turned out Arthur had other problems that the prism lenses had corrected. Reading was challenging and he had difficulty with depth perception. He was a practicing ENT physician, and as he cared for his patients, he realized that many of them who were suffering with dizziness and headache and did not have a problem with their inner ear (as their inner ear testing had been normal). As he listened more closely to their histories, it dawned on him that they were having symptoms similar to what he had experienced. Could it be that they had an eye alignment problem too? So he started sending his dizzy patients to Dr. Debby. They started to improve. She couldn't believe it because they were discouraged in school from even taking the measurements – they were hard to interpret, and they were difficult to use to make adjustments to the lens prescription. Her Dad, Dr. Paul C. Feinberg, whose office she went into had always insisted that she take those measurements when she was a new graduate otherwise she would never have found the vertical misalignment in Arthur or the patients he sent her. In school, they were taught that eye misalignment could cause eye pain and maybe headache and some challenges with reading but they were never taught it could cause other problems. Like migraines, dizziness, vertigo, motion sickness, nausea, drifting while walking, problems with balance and coordination, falling, anxiety, agoraphobia, panic attacks, suicidal ideation, overwhelmed in crowds or malls, neck pain, dyslexia, words moving on the page, skipping lines, difficulty with comprehension. It is hard to believe that these problems that people are weighed down with can be fixed with prisms added to their glasses. Did I mention that most agoraphobics have 20/20 vision? I had all my life until I needed reading glasses when I got over 50. Don't use your eye exam to prove you don't have this. Dr. Debby Feinberg also wrote a book and in it she tells her story and the story of the patients she has helped. The name of the book is "IF THE WALLS OF MY EXAM ROOM COULD TALK" By Debby Feinberg O.D.

Let's get on with the test to see if you fit into the above category. I know you are anxious to take it.

On a separate sheet of paper write the answers down.

After you take the test you can grade it.
Always= 3 points
Frequently= 2 points
Occasionally =1 points
Never =0 points

A score of 15 points or higher could mean you are a candidate for this.

Directions: For each of the following questions, please check the answer that best describes your situation. If you wear glasses or contact lenses, answer the questions assuming that you are wearing them. Please answer every question.

Never = Never
Occasionally=Less than 1 time / week
Frequently= At least 1time/ week
Always= Everyday

1. Do you have headaches and /or facial pain?
   Never
   Occasionally
   Frequently
   Always

2. Do you have pain in your eyes with eye movement?
   Never
   Occasionally
   Frequently
   Always

3. Do you experience neck or shoulder discomfort?
   Never
   Occasionally
   Frequently
   Always

4. Do you have dizziness and / or lightheadedness?
   Never
   Occasionally
   Frequently
   Always

5. Do you experience dizziness, light-headedness, or nausea while performing close-up activities (i.e. - computer work, reading, writing)?
    Never
    Occasionally
    Frequently
    Always

6. Do you experience dizziness, light-headedness, or nausea while performing far-distance activities (i.e. - driving, television, movies)?
    Never
    Occasionally
    Frequently
    Always

7. Do you experience dizziness, light-headedness, or nausea when bending down and standing back up, or when getting up quickly from a seated position?
    Never
    Occasionally
    Frequently
    Always

8. Do you feel unsteady with walking, or drift to one side while walking?

Never

Occasionally

Frequently

Always

9. Do you feel overwhelmed or anxious while walking in a large department store (i.e. – Target, Wal-Mart, Meijer)?

Never

Occasionally

Frequently

Always

10. Do you feel overwhelmed or anxious when in a crowd?

Never

Occasionally

Frequently

Always

11. Does riding in a car make you feel dizzy or uncomfortable?

Never

Occasionally

Frequently

Always

12. Do you experience anxiety or nervousness because of your dizziness?
	Never
	Occasionally
	Frequently
	Always

13. Do you ever find yourself with your head tilted to one side?
	Never
	Occasionally
	Frequently
	Always

14. Do you experience poor depth perception or have difficulty estimating distances accurately?
	Never
	Occasionally
	Frequently
	Always

15. Do you experience double / overlapping / shadowed vision at far distances?
	Never
	Occasionally
	Frequently
	Always

16. Do you experience double / overlapping / shadowed vision at near distances?
    Never
    Occasionally
    Frequently
    Always

17. Do you experience glare or have sensitivity to bright lights?
    Never
    Occasionally
    Frequently
    Always

18. Do you close or cover one eye with near or far tasks?
    Never
    Occasionally
    Frequently
    Always

19. Do you skip lines or lose your place while reading (do you use your finger or a ruler or other guides to maintain your position on the page)?
    Never
    Occasionally
    Frequently
    Always

20. Do you tire easily with close-up tasks (computer work, reading, writing)?
    Never
    Occasionally
    Frequently
    Always

21. Do you experience blurred vision with far-distance activities (i.e. - driving, television, movies, chalkboard at school)?
    Never
    Occasionally
    Frequently
    Always

22. Do you experience blurred vision with close-up activities (i.e. - computer work, reading, writing)?
    Never
    Occasionally
    Frequently
    Always

23. Do you blink to "clear up" distant objects after working at a desk or working with close-up activities (i.e. - computer work, reading, writing)?
    Never
    Occasionally
    Frequently
    Always

24. Do you experience words running together with reading?
    Never
    Occasionally
    Frequently
    Always

25. Do you experience difficulty with reading or reading comprehension?
    Never
    Occasionally
    Frequently
    Always

I also have another test for you to take. This is a cover test to be done when you are in the height of a symptom or panic. This test should reduce your symptoms. If this is the case, you can know for sure you probably need prism glasses because your condition is your eyes.

5-Minute Cover Test

1. If you have glasses or contact lenses that you wear normally for distance vision, wear them for this test

2. Determine what symptom you are most bothered by on a daily basis

  a. Write down your symptom level at this moment on a scale of 0-10.

  b. If you are not experiencing symptoms at this time you cannot do this test until you are experiencing symptoms

3. Get a timing device (phone, kitchen timer, etc.).

4. Sit down somewhere comfortable

5. Keep both eyes open and "casually glance" out 8-10 feet, covering one eye

  a. Try to refrain from looking at any particular patterns

  b. Do not text or use the computer during this test

  c. Place your timer on for 5 minutes

6. At the end of the 5 minutes, before uncovering your eye, determine on a scale of 0-10 the level of your symptom

  a. Write down the symptom level and compare to your previous symptom level

7. If you don't know which eye you should cover, do the cover test for each eye with a 20-minute period in between each eye.

  a. (Repeat steps 5-6 with 20 minutes in between each eye)

Here is a list of doctors that are currently using the Dr. Debby Feinberg method:

Vision Specialists of Michigan: Dr. Debby Feinberg, 2550 Telegraph Road, Suite #100 Bloomfield Hills MI 48302 Phone 248-258-9000 Fax 248-499-6372

Cheryl Israeloff, O.D. 300 Garden City Plaza Suite 404, Garden City, NY 11530
Phone 516-302-4053

Vince Penza, O.D. City Optometry 530 Bush St. #101, San Francisco, Ca 94108 Phone:4152918560

Neurovision Rehabilitation Center of PA, 1170 Erbs Quarry Rd. Suite4, Lititz, PA 17543

David Blair, O.D. Primary Eye Care Associates, 1821 Florence Pike, Suite 1 Burlington, KY 41005

James Aversa, O.D. 227 Boulevard, Hasbrouck Heights, NJ 07604 Phone: 2012881109

Our Vision Center, 5630 W. Dempster St. Morton Grove, Illinois 60053 Phone: 8475811891

I See Vision Care, 6651 Woolbright Road, Suite 112, Boynton Beach, Florida 33437 Phone:5617339008

Fox Chase Family Eye Care, 7834 Oxford Avenue, Philadelphia, PA 19111

Family Eyecare Center, 7500 Ramble Way, Suite 101, Raleigh, NC 27616-4310

Ithaca Eye Care Optometry, 414 E. Upland Rd. Suite A, Ithaca, NY 14850

Clark Eye Care Center, 4314 Kemp Blvd. Wichita Falls, TX 76308

Sorry there aren't more names than these but thanks to these brave pioneers there could be help in your neck of the woods. A plea is going out to more doctors to join the ones above. Call Vision Specialists to see how you could learn this important method and help your fellow man. Since I started this book Dr. Hong became the first doctor doing the Feinberg method in Illinois. I can't believe my good fortune. Thank you, Dr. Hong. Now you have all the information you need to get started. I am going to tell you the ins and outs of what you should do to complete your recovery now that you're on your way.

First let's talk about what Agoraphobia isn't.

Agoraphobia is not a mental illness. I am sorry to have to inform you that you are not nuts. You might be a little quirky but so are a lot of us. The World Health Organization and the American Psychiatric Association say that the word mental illness and neurological disorder are tossed about. The words Mental Disorder and Mental Illness are a source of contention. They can't figure out how to apply them and to what.

At one time homosexuality was listed in the DSM as mental illness but was removed when the American Psychiatric Association officially stated that homosexuality per se implies no impairment in judgment, stability, reliability or general social or vocational capabilities.

We have been told we need a psychiatrist to talk about our childhood and what was done to us. Let's face it everybody had something going on in their childhood. Some more traumatic than others. With this theory you fall into the victim mentality and never get better. It's so much easier to blame someone else.

The Medical Community has their machines. The MRI, the Cat Scan and any other contrivance they can find but the end result is always the same "can't find anything wrong with you".

Let's discuss another misconception: Serotonin levels in the brain and SSRI'S!

It's important to remember that SSRI drugs such as Prozac, Zoloft, Paxil, Lexapro, do not raise the level of Serotonin in the brain. Rather they work by Inhibiting the reuptake of Serotonin that already exists in the brain, thus resulting in a slightly higher buildup of Serotonin to remain in stasis between the billions of receptors in the brain. This inhibition of reuptake allows for improved brain functioning as it relates to mood and wellbeing because more Serotonin is left in stasis between the receptors of the brain that rely on this presence of Serotonin to properly fire. Think of it like a tiny bit of fuel in between two slightly spaced apart receptors. The receptors need this Serotonin as a kind of bridge to fire data back and forth. When the Serotonin is artificially (with meds) prevented from being absorbed by the brain, more of it can stay in the little places between the receptors to do what it does best, act as a bridge for firing data to different parts of the brain.

To take any drug that is designed to increase the amount of Serotonin in the brain is very dangerous. These drugs do exist. For example, the drug Ecstasy does this very well.

The problem with taking a drug that directly pumps Extra Serotonin into the brain is that eventually your body will do what it does best. It will stop naturally producing Serotonin because it is getting it artificially. For this to happen would be a nightmare scenario and could result in eventual brain damage. I take Xanax only and when I need it because these drugs can be habit forming both the SSRI' S and the benzodiazepines. Ok, now that we have all that straight I'm going to tell you my journey through the nightmare of agoraphobia and into the quiet and peace of real life. Huh! Did I just say that? I mean the reality that other people consider real life.

It has been about 9 years since my AH- HA moment in the shower and my first visit to Vision Specialists of Michigan. I had taken the on-line test and found to be a candidate for vertical Heterophoria. I was so confident that the minute I put on the prism glasses I would be totally fine I told my husband I would drive back from Michigan. It was a 6-hour drive but I was that convinced my whole life would change the moment I put my new glasses on. Not only did that not happen but I didn't even come home with my glasses. My first visit lasted 8 hours. Let me tell you how this is not like a regular eye doctor exam. The office comes equipped with hot tea and other hot and cold drinks plus snacks to get you through. That was nine years ago so I don't think it takes that long any more. I was even sent out on a field trip, (this does not happen to everyone.) After you are tested you are fitted with temporary prism glasses to see how you do. I was sent out on this field trip to see if I could tell a difference. Because this is a new way of looking at eyes and physical conditions you should not expect the normal eye exam you are used to. We spent 3 days in Michigan. Needless to say, I did not drive home. You should know that this condition is considered a medical condition and your exam should be covered by your health insurance and Medicare.

We were told that the glasses would be sent to me, so back home we went and I patiently waited for their arrival.

One day in the mail there they were. I put them on and instantly had double vision. After calling the office they told me to bring them back and don't wear them. One month later up to Michigan we went and I had a new vision test and new glasses. This time I did not have double vision but I wasn't any different than before. So we waited another month and went back and adjustments were made. Expecting a bigger improvement than I was getting was a disappointment. Dr. Debby knew I was about to give up. I definitely was becoming discouraged. I also had gone off Xanax that I had taken for over 20 years, the thinking being I would see improvement faster. She looked me in the eyes and said" we don't give up on anyone" Whew! That was what I needed to hear, so with renewed hope we went home.

I must tell you it was about this time that Dr. Debby talked about a head tilt and if I looked at pictures of myself I would be able to tell if I had this. After looking at the pictures I couldn't believe it, my head was almost flat. Not just in one picture but in everyone. This knowledge made a big difference in my treatment. She also told me to write in a notebook every little thing that I thought was different in my world and how I saw it. After being told to look for these things I started noticing things being different. While out in the back yard (about the furthest I could go without symptoms) I started noticing the trees seemed closer. When we went to the store I could get further back in the store without feeling anxious, and the front door didn't seem as far away. I had to be right beside my husband hanging on to the cart to even get through the store. As I am writing this I am starting to forget some of the things I couldn't do then. As hard as it is to believe I really did start to feel different. Not all people are the same. Some people get relief right away others don't. Of course I had to be the one who didn't. Dr. Debby told me I would have to find the new normal. She wasn't kidding, it wasn't instantaneous I would say over a period of about 2 months' things started to change. I was now 69 years old and had agoraphobia since I was 28. That is one of the reasons I am writing this book to let you know the sooner you start the better you will be.

It's important that you know that prisms are put into your glasses a little at a time. You cannot put all the correction in at once or you would be worse than when you started, that is the reason for all the visits until you come to a place you feel comfortable. Hopefully you have seen at least an 80% lessening of your symptoms.

My first big test! Stephanie my granddaughter was graduating from high school and she wanted us to be there, but there was just one little problem my daughter and son in law lived in California! Now we had been there before but we always took the train which wasn't easy either. The first few train trips were ok but I was just tired of putting up with all the hassle. My husband said do you want to go by train or fly. FLY? I had never flown before. I had to think that one over, maybe I could do this I wasn't completely against the idea, I decided to fly. To say this was out of my comfort zone is the understatement of all time. My biggest problem was walking through the airport. That is O'Hare airport in Chicago. I was picturing me standing in line in this big open space. Remember we don't do open spaces. By this time, I was doing open spaces a lot better than I ever had before so my courage was up a bit. We arrived at the airport and made it to our gate without much trouble. It helped that I had a neighbor who worked there and was kind enough to help us through. The flight is over 4 hours but it was a piece of cake compared to the train that was 2 nights and 3 days. It was really exciting going down the runway and lifting off.

Now the next big hurdle was sitting in the massive crowd in the stadium where she was graduating. The thought of people sitting in back of me sent me crazy. The only good thing was that it was outside. After sitting down, I started looking for an escape route, that's the first thing agoraphobics do. The graduation started and before I could work up a good dizzy pitching forth spell it was over and I was fine. I couldn't believe it. Not one bit of panic ever came near me. Confidence in my prism glasses skyrocketed after that.

Did I mention that I had been seeing a psychiatrist for about 25 years by then? I told him I was going to fly to California and he said that people who have what I have couldn't do that. By the time I had done it over 3 times he changed his mind. I tried to get him to tell his patients about Dr. Debby and Vision Specialists of Michigan but he wouldn't. The medical profession is very slow to accept new ideas. Take Vitamin C for example. After it was found out that scurvy is caused by a lack of vitamin C it took the medical community 400 years to accept it! Hard to believe but true. I told my psychiatrist I was going to write a book and he was thrilled but shortly after that he died of cancer, he was ten years younger than me. I like to think he eventually would have accepted Vertical Heterophoria as the cause of Agoraphobia and bring this knowledge to his patients. I liked him very much.

It is now time to talk about the" D" word. D for desensitization. The first time I came anywhere near this word was many years ago when I first came down with agoraphobia. A psychologist that I went to see had a plan to get me back into the car. He had two walkie talkies, I had one he had the other. The plan was for him to follow me in the car and when I was feeling panicky I could talk to him and he would talk me out of it. To make a very long story short I headed for home after 30 minutes of total panic and didn't recoup for 3 days. I was in total shell shock. After that disaster I was referred to a psychiatrist and put on meds. Now after saying all that the biggest part of your recovery will be DESENSITIZATION!

The one thing we cannot do is put the cart before the horse. That is what they are doing in the current methods of desensitization. That is like telling the person without a leg to just run anyway and they will forget the fact they don't have a leg. First we put the artificial leg on and then we learn to walk and then run. In our case we first have an eye exam with an optometrist that is schooled in the neuro visual medical field (refer to the ones I have listed here.) You will be fitted with a pair of prism glasses even if you have 20/20 vision. One visit might not be enough. I was the one who decided if I needed another appointment. I am not sure how it is being done today. After you start feeling some relief you start the desensitization. The glasses are your artificial leg now you can practice becoming well. Remember prisms are put in a little at a time. Easy does it.

In my case I would need to go grocery shopping every week or sometimes we would go to the store for something or other. We went to Wal-Mart a lot. For best results starting out, go with someone until you start feeling comfortable. You will need your safe person for a while. I have to tell you one of my Wal-Mart stories. I would go into the store and hang onto my cart like it was an extension of my body. My hand never came off of the handle. If I wanted to look at something I would keep a hand on the cart while looking. I noticed that if I walked down the aisle fast I would be dizzy. Mostly I would shop the grocery section and looking at the shelf was a blur of different colors whizzing by. So I would just slow down until the dizzy passed. Now if you're like me the one thing we like to do it "getter done." We do everything fast. Remember the NEW NORMAL? You have to learn to slow down. This can take a while but have patience it will happen. Don't rush yourself take your time and notice everything that is happening to you, the good, bad and the ugly. Everyone is different so I cannot give you a time frame when you will start to notice but you will notice.

Another story I remember really well is again at Wal-Mart, I am going down the aisle and all of a sudden I feel like I am at an angle, my whole body is off to the right, this was kind of scary but I just told myself this must be part of getting used to the glasses. So, while I was in the store I would never know what was going to happen, but believing whatever it was I was getting better helped. I just had to get used to these new feelings.

The first time I could stand in a wide-open space and did not feel dizzy, like I was pitching forward was a real revelation, I couldn't believe it. My husband was retired so I called him my girlfriend we went everywhere together which made my recovery easier. Eventually I quit hanging on the cart and now when we go to the store I take one cart and my husband takes another and we meet at the vegetables. I didn't need him anymore to go up and down the aisles. I would say it took a good 2 years for this to happen. It could happen faster for you. Remember I have had this for over 40 years. I had more time feeling bad than good in my life.

Sometimes I would feel the old feeling of panic and dizzy coming on and I would adjust my glasses and it would go away, or wait a few minutes and it would just go.

Especially if I was talking to a lot of people I would keep moving my head and the dizzy would come over me. You will learn the things you can and can't do. Eventually you recognize the symptoms and adjust for them. Remember you have a physical disability the prism glasses are helping you live with it. There is no magic pill to take and make it all go away because you were born this way. You have to accept that and go on with your life. Once you properly become desensitized you will never have a relapse. The only direction for you will be forward, I promise you. Dr Debby promises you a reduction of your symptoms about 80%. My reduction was about 90 to 95%. The important thing is for your mind to forget your awful past with ago-raphobia symptoms and to become accustomed to your new life without them. I have another story to tell you.

I moved about 4 years ago. When I walked into my closet in the old house the light switch was on the inside of the door, in my new house it is on the outside. When my mind is busy somewhere else I walk into the closet and look for the switch inside. In 4 years my mind has not forgotten the old house. That is why it is so important to get help immediately.

Things I couldn't conquer completely. ANXIETY is an ongoing thing, not anything like it was but when I start to do things that I just couldn't do before the anxiety starts in but very mild compared to before the prism glasses.

Driving is something I do but I am never very comfortable with it. It kind of makes sense if you think the car is not only in a big open space but there are lines on the right and left you have to stay between. All the triggers for an agoraphobia event. I even still have trouble riding in a car. Actually it all depends on who is driving. If I don't trust the driver I am really anxious. This year I had to take a driving test for a new driving license. I worried for over a year. I am 77 years old so I thought maybe I should just quit. After all it wouldn't seem weird at my age if I said I'm done. But I keep trying not to look at my age. Otherwise I will start giving myself a pass all the time. After I passed and got my license I realized that all the old people are in the same boat. Once you hit a certain age it is mandatory. The lady before me had the Driving Examiner put her walker in the back seat while she got into the driver's seat. Being old has some advantages. This accomplishment was almost as big as flying in the airplane. Before you know it, you will realize that people without agoraphobia have all the same anxious feelings you have, especially about going for a driving test.

SPONTANEITY is another thing I couldn't conquer. I can't just run out the door get in my car and go. I have to have a heads up that I need to do something. It still takes me time to think about it. I just don't get worked up any more. I went from home bound to pretty much normal.

My personality started to change. I started feeling one with people, not like I used to feel and think. In the past, it was always how can I hide my problem from whoever I was interacting with, now with the problem solved I didn't even think that way and started enjoying being with people and listening to them. I became a kinder person. I really liked the new me.

After having gone through all of this I found out the name of another problem I have always had and it is Monophobia! This is the fear of being alone. I mainly don't like being alone at night. This has been something I have had all my life. Glasses won't fix this. Once your agoraphobia is gone you might find you have other things also. The only thing I know for sure, the prism glasses will definitely get rid of your agoraphobia because that is not a mental problem but phobias are, maybe one day the cause of those will be realized.

Thinking about me all the time when I left the house was fading away. Before the glasses I could not sit in an audience, because I felt everyone was looking at me not to mention the dizzy pitching forward feeling. Now I felt more like we were there for the same reason. My feelings of people looking at me were gone. I started to listen to people because now I didn't have to worry that I was going to pass out or fall over. People were very interesting! The little bonuses keep adding up. It was wonderful. I didn't feel like my neck was on a hinge and my head would fall off at any minute. It is hard to believe that a simple pair of prism glasses could change my whole world.

Not many people knew I had agoraphobia. After I wrote my first book people who knew me just wouldn't believe that I had any of that. My own husband included.

They said I just wrote the book to get something off my chest. My personality is very outgoing, truly I was a closet agoraphobic. I went to great lengths to hide my disability. Now I talk about it much more, I actually feel comfortable talking about it. I have a blog at "agoraphobiawhat. blogspot.com" when I first started this blog I wouldn't post to Facebook because I knew too many people there, but one day I just said "I really don't care what people think about me. If this will help somebody I have to do it".

It is hard for our family's to accept this in us. There are people with PHD's and Masters that can't leave their homes. A lot of talent is lost to agoraphobia. Just the loss of self-worth is overwhelming. There are those that abuse drugs and alcohol to be able to live in this world. Agoraphobics are all over the world, in every race in every color. It shouldn't be this way. IT'S YOUR EYES! I hope you will listen and then tell everyone you know the answer is simple, because it is.

Maybe we should talk about medication. I take Xanax as needed, I could go as long as four days without a Xanax and then again I might need one every day for a week. I am very careful not to increase the dosage because it is habit forming. I take high blood pressure medicine so why not something for anxiety? Don't beat yourself up for having to take medication. Just be careful that you do not increase the dosage. You will find the prism glasses work better than any medication.

I would like to say a few things about Attention Deficit Disorder or ADD. This can also be caused by Binocular Vision Dysfunction. Some of the symptoms are

Tilt of the head
Motion sickness
Nausea/Difficulty gaining weight
Clumsiness (poor depth perception)
Headaches
Dizziness
Sore, tired eyes
Skipped lines when reading
Re-reading for comprehension
Blurred or double vision
Light sensitivity
Closing or covering an eye
Anxiety

Eye tests do not find BVD in school, so if you suspect your child could have this instead of medicating maybe a pair of prism glasses fitted by a specialist in this field would be the answer. I can only recommend the eye doctors listed here.

This is the end of my story. I hope you have found some useful information in these pages. Please talk to someone you know who has agoraphobia and tell them about this book and the prism glasses.

A Special Thank you to Dr. Paul Feinberg for teaching his daughter that not everything is learned in school and to Dr. Debbie Feinberg for listening to that advise and being the pioneer in the field of Vertical Heterophoria or BVD.

I wish you all the best as you struggle through life because life is meant to be a struggle so we can become better. Just remember it is about the LOVE you demonstrate to your fellow man that God sees.

Love and Hugs, Yolanda